Get Through MRCPsych Parts 1 and 2:
525 Individual Statement Questions in Psychopathology

Get Through MRCPsych Parts 1 and 2: 525 Individual Statement Questions in Psychopathology

Juan Antonio Retamero LMS MRCPsych

Senior House Officer in Psychiatry
Guy's King's and St Thomas' Training Scheme, Princess Royal Hospital,
Haywards Heath, West Sussex

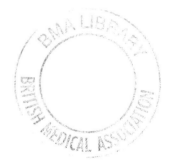

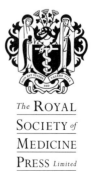

The ROYAL
SOCIETY *of*
MEDICINE
PRESS *Limited*

©2006 Royal Society of Medicine Ltd

Published by the Royal Society of Medicine Press Ltd
1 Wimpole Street, London W1G 0AE, UK
Tel: +44 (0)20 7290 2921
Fax: +44 (0)20 7290 2929
E-mail: publishing@rsmpress.co.uk

British Library Cataloguing in Publication Data
A catalogue record for this book is available from the British Library

ISBN: 1-85315-608-6

Distribution in Europe and Rest of the World:

Marston Book Services Ltd
PO Box 269
Abingdon
Oxon OX14 4YN, UK
Tel: +44 (0)1235 465500
Fax: +44 (0)1235 465555
Email: direct.order@marston.co.uk

Distribution in USA and Canada:

Royal Society of Medicine Press Ltd
c/o BookMasters Inc
30 Amberwood Parkway
Ashland, OH 44805, USA
Tel: +1 800 247 6553/+1 800 266 5564
Fax: +1 419 281 6883
Email: orders@bookmasters.com

Distribution in Australia and New Zealand:

Elsevier Australia
30–52 Smidmore Street
Marrikville NSW 2204, Australia
Tel: +61 2 9517 8999
Fax: +61 2 9517 2249
Email: service@elsevier.com.au

Phototypeset by Phoenix Photosetting, Chatham, Kent
Printed in the UK by Bell & Bain Ltd, Glasgow

Contents

Preface

Psychopathology can be defined as the study of abnormal experience and behaviour. It constitutes the 'bread and butter' for the psychiatrist, and is no less important in other associated professions. This fact is reflected in the MRCPsych examination, as psychopathology is one of the most frequent topics covered in the written components of both parts of the examination.

This book is mainly aimed at junior psychiatrists preparing for part one of the MRCPsych examination, but it will also be helpful to those preparing for part two. It will also be helpful for psychologists, psychiatric nurses, social workers and other mental health professionals in contact with patients who wish to refresh their knowledge in this topic. My intention in writing this book was to introduce the topic by tapping into the knowledge that the mental health professional already possesses in psychopathology, and progressively enhancing it. It should be an ideal revision tool for those sitting the MRCPsych examination, but it has also been written for the junior doctor who may have just started psychiatric training.

This book contains 525 individual statement questions in psychopathology, divided into five papers. The first part of each paper comprises the questions and the second half contains the answers. I have added additional comments to some answers in order to clarify and expand the reader's understanding in that area. The questions are generally grouped in different topics, and their level of difficulty is gradually increased within each topic. The topics that I have selected in this book are those most frequently asked in the Royal College of Psychiatrists' examinations. I believe that this is an effective way not only to learn the minutiae of the many concepts covered, but also to help to revise a topic already covered.

I would recommend that the reader should try to answer every question in sequence, making a note of the answers, and then check the answer section, paying attention to the explanations and comments given.

This book is dedicated to my wife, Navidad, and our baby son, Jaime, as a sign of gratitude for their patience and support. I should also like to show my gratitude to Senior Consultant Psychiatrist Ayaz Begg for reviewing all of the questions in the book.

Finally, I hope that this book will help the reader gain a better understanding of this fascinating subject, and that this may be useful to comprehend better the experiences of those with mental illness.

Juan A Retamero

Paper 1
Questions

Paper 1
Questions

1. Narcolepsy is associated with hyperphagia.

2. Classification systems in psychiatry are usually based on description of symptoms.

3. Somatic hallucinations are first rank symptoms.

4. Disorientation for place in delirium tremens indicates development of Wernicke's syndrome.

5. Anhedonia can be reliably assessed using a questionnaire.

6. In diagnosis, the form of a subjective experience is more important than the content.

7. Catalepsy occurs in narcolepsy.

8. Perseveration suggests a functional illness rather than dementia.

9. Classification of symptoms in psychiatry is usually based on pathological findings.

10. The international personality disorder examination (IPDE) is routinely used in clinical practice.

11. Musical hallucinations in peripheral deafness indicate psychosis.

12. Inquiring about suicidal intention may provoke it and should, therefore, be discouraged.

13. Waxy flexibility is rarely seen in schizophrenia.

14. Loosening of associations is key in differentiating mania from schizophrenia.

15. Anhedonia seldom occurs in schizophrenia.

16. Visual hallucinations are seen in more than 30% of schizophrenics.

17. Waxy flexibility is a plastic resistance to gentle movement.

Paper I
Questions

18. ICD-10 states that delusions and hallucinations should not dominate the picture in hebephrenic schizophrenia.

19. Delusional perception can be secondary to auditory hallucinations.

20. Negativism is part of the cognitive syndrome in depression.

21. Delusional perception is a delusion that is formed after a normal perception.

22. Anhedonia is often seen in psychotic depression.

23. Pareidolia is a common feature of schizophrenia.

24. Pareidolia is seen in normal people.

25. Elementary hallucinations can include hearing voices.

26. Obsessional thoughts are recognised as senseless.

27. Anhedonia is a psychopathological symptom that implies a limited range of negative emotions.

28. Anhedonia is frequently seen in depressive states.

29. Anhedonia is synonymous with inability to experience pleasure.

30. The term anhedonia relates to the loss of ability to experience pleasure.

31. The presence of anhedonia is essential to differentiate between psychotic depression and schizophrenia.

32. Night terrors occur in post-traumatic stress disorder (PTSD).

33. Derealisation is a change in the awareness of the external world.

34. Hallucinations can occur in normal people.

35. Klein introduced the term anhedonia, stating that it is the best clinical marker for predicting response to treatment in depressive illness.

Paper I
Questions

36. A patient who does not complain of depressed mood cannot be, by definition, depressed.

37. The term melancholic figures in DSM-IV in relation to depression.

38. Anhedonia can be described as the complete inability to experience pleasure.

39. Retardation is the slowing down of the ability to think or act, and it is usually associated with self-blame and reduced self-esteem.

40. According to Kraepelin, the depressed patient can have a negative view of himself and his ongoing experiences, and has a negative view of the future.

41. A patient who complains of total lack of interest in his normal hobbies suffers from anhedonia.

42. Anhedonia is a passivity phenomenon.

43. Depersonalisation involves a change in the awareness of the self.

44. Depersonalisation is an 'as if' experience where the individual feels 'unreal'.

45. Depersonalisation is a rather uncommon phenomenon in the psychiatric setting.

46. Depersonalisation can be pleasurable and enjoyable, particularly when associated with the use of certain psychoactive substances.

47. In most cases of depersonalisation, insight is lost.

48. Phantom limb is a dissociative phenomenon.

49. There is always a change in mood associated with depersonalisation.

50. Depersonalisation and derealisation are commonly seen together.

51. The loss of ego boundaries seen in schizophrenia is defined as depersonalisation.

Paper I
Questions

52. Loosening of associations and derailment are phenomenologically unrelated terms.

53. In pure depersonalisation, there can be a component of delusional elaboration.

54. Emotional numbing has been described as part of the myriad of symptoms related to depersonalisation.

55. Depersonalisation can be associated with changes in any perceptual modality.

56. Depersonalisation is a functional symptom, and it is absent in organic states.

57. Depersonalisation and derealisation are frequently experienced together.

58. Depersonalisation is rarely associated with an unpleasant emotion.

59. Depersonalisation and derealisation, by definition, do not occur in the absence of psychiatric illness.

60. Derealisation and depersonalisation are, on most occasions, easy to distinguish from each other.

61. Depersonalisation is related to anxiety.

62. Phobic symptoms are often agoraphobic in nature.

63. Agoraphobia is most common amongst married females in their thirties.

64. Depersonalisation and derealisation appear in ICD-10 as a separate nosologic entity.

65. Depersonalisation and derealisation can be both symptoms and syndromes.

66. The majority of patients affected agree that derealisation is straightforward to describe.

5

Paper I
Questions

67. Depersonalisation affects the patient's outer space, and derealisation is its equivalent in the inner space.

68. The feeling of familiarity normally associated with the perception of the self is lost in depersonalisation.

69. Depersonalisation may occur in cannabis intoxication.

70. The change of awareness of self and its surroundings present in depersonalisation is always unpleasant to the subject.

71. Desomatisation is closely associated with depersonalisation.

72. Desomatisation is a key feature in koro.

73. Déjà vu and depersonalisation share an alteration in the sense of familiarity associated with perceptions of the environment and the self, respectively.

74. The experience of depersonalisation rarely lasts longer than a few seconds.

75. Depersonalisation can appear in cases of PTSD.

76. Depersonalisation occurs linked to dissociation in the majority of cases.

77. Derealisation cannot be induced.

78. Depersonalisation and derealisation are usually described amongst patients in a manic or hypomanic phase in the context of bipolar affective disorder.

79. Some parallelism has been established between depersonalisation and ecstasy.

80. Dizziness has been described as sharing a common ground with depersonalisation.

81. Depersonalisation can be experienced by normal people.

82. True delusion and primary delusion are synonymous.

83. Primary delusions occur more frequently in acute rather than chronic schizophrenia.

84. Only secondary delusions deserve the epithet of true delusions.

85. Schneider's first rank symptoms usually point out the primary source of psychopathological symptomatology.

86. Perception of time is altered in depersonalisation.

87. Primary delusions are a Schneiderian first rank symptom.

88. Delusion-like ideas can be understood in the context of the patient's state.

89. Delusion-like ideas and delusional perception are equivalent terms.

90. Primary delusions are characterised by being psychologically irreducible.

91. Schneider described three types of true or primary delusions: autochthonous delusion (delusional intuition), delusional percept and delusional memory.

92. A delusional intuition typically appears following an autochthonous delusion.

93. Autochthonous delusions typically occur in one single stage.

94. Wahneinfall and delusional perception are equivalent terms.

95. A delusional intuition cannot be differentiated by the subject from a normal idea.

96. A delusional percept is a normal percept that is given a delusional meaning, usually with great personal significance.

97. A delusional percept is a first rank symptom of schizophrenia.

98. A delusional perception is characterised by the abnormal significance attached to a normal perception.

Paper I
Questions

99. Secondary delusions are synonymous with delusion-like ideas.

100. Delusional perceptions are, by definition, those abnormal ideas that arise from a hallucinatory experience.

101. A delusional perception is a two-step process whereby an abnormal perception is given a delusional meaning that is usually of the greatest importance to the patient.

102. In phenomenological terms, it is appropriate to conclude that a delusional perception is a simple interpretation of a normal perception.

103. In delusional perception, there is a normal perception associated with a meaningful delusional explanation of that perception.

104. In delusional perception, delusional meaning can be given to any sensation, in any modality.

105. In delusional perception, an abnormal meaning is attached to a normal perception almost immediately after being perceived.

Paper 1
Answers

Paper I
Answers

1. True. They are seen together in the Kleine–Levin syndrome, which involves episodes of somnolence and increased appetite that can last for weeks, with long intervals in between attacks.

2. True.

3. False.

4. False.

5. True.

6. True.

7. False. Cataplexy is a sudden loss of muscular tone, and occurs in narcolepsy. Catalepsy refers to motor disorders typically seen in schizophrenia.

8. False. Perseveration is quite suggestive of an organic process. It is typically associated with clouding of consciousness and involves issuing a response that is appropriate to a first stimulus, but it is repeated inappropriately on a second stimulus.

9. False.

10. False.

11. False.

12. False.

13. True.

14. False. Loosening of associations appears in both conditions.

15. False.

16. False.

17. True.

18. True.

Paper 1
Answers

19. False.

20. False. Negativism is characterised by a persistent opposition and resistance to suggestions.

21. True.

22. True.

23. False.

24. True. Pareidolia involves seeing concrete figures in abstract shapes, using a certain degree of imagination. It is a normal phenomenon, although it can be induced by psychomimetic drugs.

25. False.

26. True.

27. False.

28. True.

29. True.

30. True. Ribot introduced the term in 1896.

31. False.

32. False.

33. True.

34. True.

35. False. Klein saw it as such, but Ribot coined the term.

36. False. The term 'depressio sine depressione' can be used in those patients who present with other features of depression without complaining of depressed mood.

Paper I
Answers

37. True. Melancholic depression is characterised by the presence of biological (somatic) features, such as psychomotor retardation, early morning wakening, diurnal variation of mood, poor appetite and weight loss.

38. True.

39. True.

40. False. This is Beck's cognitive triad.

41. True.

42. False.

43. True.

44. True.

45. False. It can occur in up to 30% of all new out-patient referrals.

46. False. It is always unpleasant.

47. False.

48. False.

49. True.

50. True.

51. False.

52. False. They are quite closely related, and it can be difficult to differentiate one from the other.

53. False.

54. True.

55. True.

56. False. It can be present in organic states, especially temporal lobe epilepsy and cannabis intoxication.

57. True. This is because the ego and its surroundings are experienced as a continuum.

58. False.

59. False. It can be experienced by normal people, although typically appears in depression and dissociative states.

60. False.

61. True.

62. True.

63. True.

64. True. See ICD–10 F48.1

65. True.

66. False.

67. False. It is the other way round.

68. True.

69. True.

70. True.

71. True. It is the alteration of the sense of familiarity normally associated with an individual organ.

72. True. Koro denotes a state of transient anxiety in which the person is concerned about a shrinking of the penis that will result in death. First described by Yap (1965).

73. True.

74. False. It has been described to last for months.

Paper I
Answers

75. True, given the element of stress involved. It can also appear in perpetrators and victims of antisocial behaviour, sometimes accompanied with dissociation.

76. False. Although depersonalisation can be related to dissociation, it is normally associated with anxiety and depression.

77. False. Kennedy (1976) described it associated with transcendental yoga.

78. False. It tends to occur during depressive phases, but it has never been described in mania, according to Sedman (1970).

79. True. Anderson (1938) stated that one is the obverse of the other, depersonalisation occurring in depression and ecstasy in mania.

80. True. This has been proposed by Fewtrell and O'Connor.

81. True.

82. True. The first term was coined by Jaspers.

83. True.

84. False. Primary delusions are actually true delusions.

85. False. First rank symptoms are an empirical list of commonly found symptoms in schizophrenia; they do not entail any aetiological value, nor indicate prognosis. They are very helpful in confirming a diagnosis of schizophrenia. First rank symptoms are:
    - Hearing one's thoughts spoken aloud (thought echo)
    - Third person auditory hallucinations
    - Auditory hallucinations in the form of a running commentary
    - Somatic hallucinations
    - Thought withdrawal, insertion or broadcast
    - Delusional perception
    - 'Passivity phenomena'

86. True.

87. False.

88. True. Delusion-like ideas are synonymous for secondary delusion.

Paper I
Answers

89. False.

90. True.

91. False. Although the description in the question is correct, it was Jaspers who made this distinction.

92. False. Actually, these terms are synonymous.

93. True, as opposed to delusional perceptions that occur in two stages (perception and subsequent delusional interpretation).

94. True.

95. True.

96. True.

97. True.

98. True.

99. True.

100. False. They refer to the abnormal meaning that is attached to a normal perception.

101. False. Although the meaning attached to a delusional perception is very relevant to the patient, it only arises from normal perceptions.

102. False. It is a fully meaningful and relevant interpretation, of a delusional nature, of a normal experience; this means that this delusional explanation is paramount in the patient's existence.

103. True.

104. True. Usually visual perception, but it can even be formed from written words or sentences.

105. False. There can even be an interval of years between the two.

Paper 2
Questions

Paper 2
Questions

1. In delusional atmosphere, there is a typical alteration in the patient's perception of his own reality, although the patient often finds it difficult to define what this alteration involves.

2. A feeling of anticipation has been classically described associated with delusional atmosphere.

3. A delusional perception can arise in the background of delusional mood.

4. The terms delusional mood and delusional atmosphere are synonymous.

5. Delusional atmosphere is seen exclusively in schizophrenia.

6. Delusional mood is typically seen in the prodromal phases of schizophrenia.

7. Delusional atmosphere can precede delusional perception.

8. Simulation of schizophrenic symptoms can precede true schizophrenia.

9. The preservation of self-esteem is a factor involved in delusion formation.

10. Delusional memory consists of recalling an idea and investing it with delusional nature.

11. A retrospective delusion and a delusional memory are distinguishable because of their different chronology.

12. A delusional meaning that is attached to a normal percept, that is remembered, is termed a delusional memory.

13. In phenomenological terms, the distinction between delusional memory and delusional perception can be made easily on the basis of their chronological disparity.

14. By definition, a delusion is an abnormal idea of great significance to the affected patient that invariably leads him to act on it.

15. The need for consistency in the inner representation of the world is implicated in the maintenance of delusions.

16. Poverty of personal intercommunication has been involved as a contributing factor in the recovery from paranoid delusions.

17. A delusional perception involves a normal perception acquiring a new meaning.

18. A delusional perception is rarely as valuable in understanding the origin of a delusional construct as a secondary delusion.

19. The heightening of effect that Bleuler refers to as one of his primary symptoms can facilitate the loosening of associations and hence the apparition of delusions.

20. Kretschmer proposed an aetiological model for schizophrenia and other delusional illnesses where the physical appearance was the main single factor associated with the creation of delusional constructs.

21. Primary and secondary delusions differ in that secondary delusions are ultimately not understandable.

22. Eidetic imagery is a form of hallucination.

23. A delusion is a judgement that cannot be accepted by people of the same class, education, race and period of life as the person who experiences it.

24. A primary delusion is, by definition, not understandable.

25. Secondary delusions derive necessarily from primary delusions.

26. From a phenomenological point of view, there is a clear difference to the subject affected between a delusion and a normal idea.

27. Delusions are characteristically held with unusual conviction, and are not debatable to logic.

28. The term delusion is defined in ICD-10.

Paper 2
Questions

29. A visual hallucination can precede the formation of primary delusions.

30. Secondary delusions can arise following a delusional perception.

31. In general terms, it is appropriate to conclude that formal thought disorder and delusional ideas are roughly equivalent terms.

32. Delusions are typically bizarre, disorganized and involve several areas of the patient's life.

33. According to Jaspers, the main feature of primary delusions is their 'psychological irreducibility'.

34. Secondary delusions arise from other morbid phenomena and are understandable in this context.

35. A delusion that arises following a hallucinatory experience is appropriately termed secondary delusion.

36. The three main characteristics of a delusional belief are the unrivalled conviction with which they are held, the lack of amenability to logical arguments and that they are out of keeping with the person's cultural and social background.

37. Delusional mood can be followed by a primary delusion.

38. Delusions are characterised by the creation of a self-evident, private and isolating model of the world that requires no proof to be firmly believed by the sufferer.

39. Delusional atmosphere and autochthonous delusions are types of primary delusion.

40. In the aetiology of delusions, an increased awareness of irrelevant stimuli, the intrusion of unintended material from long-term memory, and an anomaly in information processing have been involved.

41. The content of delusions is normally the opposite to the prevailing mood of the patient at that time.

42. Two of the most frequent delusional themes are delusions of persecution and grandiose delusions.

43. An autochthonous delusion may follow secondary to an over-valued idea.

44. A delusional perception can arise from paranoid delusions.

45. Delusion-like ideas and secondary delusions are the same.

46. Olfactory hallucinations have been implicated in the genesis of delusional perceptions.

47. An overvalued idea is an acceptable and understandable notion that preoccupies the subject to the extent of dominating his life.

48. Overvalued ideas are mainly seen in schizophrenia and other schizophrenia-like disorders.

49. An overvalued idea is held invariably on false or erroneous grounds.

50. Overvalued ideas and obsessional thoughts are both subjectively experienced as 'senseless' by the patient.

51. Overvalued ideas are rarely acted upon.

52. Delusional perception may be preceded by delusional mood.

53. Passivity of volition is the same as made volition.

54. A person suffering from dementia has overinclusive thought.

55. In anorexia nervosa, the psychopathological substrate is usually a distortion of body image of delusional nature.

56. An overvalued idea is an acceptable idea pursued by the patient beyond the limits of reason, so it dominates the patient's life.

57. In hypochondriasis, the abnormality of thought seen is usually a delusion.

58. Transsexuals do suffer from delusional ideas related to their gender identity.

Paper 2
Questions

59. Elementary auditory hallucinations occur in alcoholic hallucinosis.

60. In paranoid personality disorder, paranoid delusions are prominent.

61. Failure to use direct questions can lead to failure to establish the severity of a mood disorder.

62. In delusional jealousy, the patient, by definition, suffers from delusional ideas.

63. In chronic alcoholism, hallucinations can be fragmentary initially.

64. In schizophrenia in learning disability, delusions can be elaborate.

65. Déjà vu is a memory disorder, in which the patient fails to associate previously lived events with current experience.

66. Déjà vu is unusually seen in schizophrenia.

67. In jamais vu, there is a lack of the associated feeling of familiarity that normally occurs with previously lived events.

68. In déjà vu, a familiar situation is experienced as totally fresh and new to the subject.

69. In jamais vu, an experience lived before by the subject is lacking the appropriate feeling of familiarity.

70. Jamais vu and déjà vu are associated with a sensation of familiarity.

71. Déjà vu is phenomenon commonly seen in schizophrenia.

72. Déjà vu can be seen in normal people.

73. In the identifying paramnesias, the appropriate feelings of familiarity associated with previously experienced situations are disturbed.

74. Phantom limb is a dissociative phenomenon.

Paper 2
Questions

75. Jamais vu is an abnormal experience that invariably denotes psychopathology.

76. Déjà vu is experienced in the aural phase of temporal lobe epilepsy.

77. In déjà vu, there is a perceived sense of familiarity around experiences not previously lived.

78. In jamais vu, an unfamiliar experience or object seems to be familiar.

79. Delusional perception is one of Schneider's first rank symptoms of schizophrenia.

80. Loosening of associations constitutes a first rank symptom.

81. Schneider described overinclusiveness among the first rank symptoms of schizophrenia.

82. Any form of auditory hallucination can be included as a first rank symptom.

83. Thought withdrawal, insertion and broadcasting are first rank symptoms of schizophrenia.

84. First rank symptoms may be commonly found in temporal lobe epilepsy.

85. Amongst first rank symptoms, Schneider included certain passivity experiences.

86. First rank symptoms are seen in affective disorders.

87. First rank symptoms are, by definition, exclusive of schizophrenia.

88. First rank symptoms constitute an exhaustive diagnostic checklist in schizophrenia.

89. The absence of first rank symptoms excludes a diagnosis of schizophrenia.

Paper 2
Questions

90. First rank symptoms are only useful in establishing a diagnosis of schizophrenia in Western cultures.

91. Paranoid delusions are a first rank symptom of schizophrenia.

92. Delusions of passivity and control are first rank symptoms.

93. The terms 'gedankenlautwerden', 'écho de pensées' and 'audible thoughts' are used as synonymous.

94. In thought insertion, there is an alteration of the boundaries of the self.

95. An individual who, during interview, claims that his ways of thinking are clearly influenced by his parent's views suffers from passivity phenomena.

96. Somatic passivity consists of the belief that foreign forces control the body.

97. The terms haptic hallucination and somatic passivity refer broadly to the same concept.

98. According to Bleuler, autism is only a secondary criterion for schizophrenia.

99. Hallucinations and delusions are considered fundamental symptoms for schizophrenia in Bleuler's classification.

100. Overinclusive thinking is one of Bleuler's primary criteria for schizophrenia.

101. Thought insertion and withdrawal are primary symptoms for schizophrenia according to Bleuler.

102. Following Bleuler's classification, catatonic phenomena are considered secondary criteria for schizophrenia.

103. Bleuler considered the presence of neologisms as a primary criterion for schizophrenia.

104. Loosening of associations, ambivalence and autism are considered of capital importance by Bleuler to establish a diagnosis of schizophrenia.

105. Thought block is a first rank symptom of schizophrenia as well as a primary criterion to Bleuler.

Paper 2
Answers

1. True.

2. True.

3. True. This is typically the case. Usually a feeling of anticipation culminates in the experience of a delusion that fills of meaning that anticipatory state.

4. True. Delusional mood is the term used in German psychopathology.

5. False. Berner considers that it can exist in other processes.

6. True.

7. True.

8. True. Particularly in people with certain deviant premorbid personalities, according to Hay (1983).

9. True. According to Brockington (1991).

10. True.

11. False. Actually, retrospective delusion and delusional memory are synonymous terms.

12. False. It is a delusional percept rather than delusional memory.

13. False. There is no absolute demarcation between delusional memory and delusional perception; the time scale is arbitrary and subjective.

14. False. Delusions are not *invariably* acted upon.

15. True.

16. False. Actually, it has been involved in the maintenance of delusions.

17. True.

Paper 2
Answers

18. False. Some authors regard delusional perception as the key to understanding delusional experience.

19. True. According to Bleuler, at the beginning of schizophrenia there is a state of increased affect that the patient finds difficult to express.

20. False. Actually Kretschmer proposed that certain personality types matched certain phenotypes; with regards to the aetiology of delusions and schizophrenia, he proposed that a sensitive premorbid personality in people who retained emotionally laden complexes was predisposed to present ideas of reference.

21. False. Secondary delusions are understandable if the primary delusions are taken into account.

22. False.

23. True. This is the definition of delusion proposed by Stoddart.

24. True. As opposed to secondary delusions that are understandable in the context of the primary psychopathological processes from which they emerge.

25. False. They can appear secondary to, for example, mood abnormalities or hallucinations.

26. False. Phenomenological here means how the affected individual perceives his own thoughts; to a delusional subject, an abnormal idea is not differentiable from a normal idea, and the difference must be established by an outsider.

27. True. The other main feature of delusions is that they are erroneous.

28. False. Although used frequently, it is not defined here.

29. False.

30. True.

31. False.

Paper 2
Answers

32. True. These dimensions of the term delusion were proposed by Kendler et al (1983). Other dimensions include conviction, pressure (in the sense of preoccupation and concern with the delusion), affective response and deviant behaviour.

33. True. This means that they appear *per se* and not in connection with any other psychopathological event.

34. True.

35. True.

36. True. This is another good definition of delusion.

37. True.

38. True.

39. True. The four different types of primary delusions are: 1) autochthonous delusions; 2) delusional perception; 3) delusional memories; and 4) delusional atmosphere. Autochthonous delusions and delusional intuitions are synonymous.

40. True.

41. False. The content of delusions is determined by the patient's personality, mood state, sociocultural background and previous experience.

42. True. Classically, six main delusional themes have been described: 1) paranoid delusions; 2) grandiose delusions; 3) delusions of guilt that may become nihilistic; 4) delusional jealousy; 5) delusions of love; and 6) hypochondriacal delusions.

43. False. Autochthonous delusions are primary delusions and, therefore, do not arise secondary to other psychopathological symptoms.

44. False.

45. True.

46. False.

Paper 2
Answers

47. True.

48. False. They are most frequent in abnormal personalities.

49. False.

50. False. Obsessional thoughts are perceived as senseless by the subject, but overvalued ideas are given the greatest importance.

51. False. They are *invariably* acted upon, like an instinct.

52. True.

53. True.

54. False.

55. False. The body image distortion is typically in the form of an overvalued idea. Other disorders with predominant overvalued ideas include: 1) morbid jealousy; 2) hypochondriasis; 3) dysmorphophobias; 4) paranoid states, as seen in paranoid personality disorder; 5) transsexualism; and 6) Ekbom syndrome (parasitophobia).

56. True.

57. False. It is typically an overvalued idea.

58. False. In transsexualism, overvalued ideas with regards to gender identity are typically present.

59. True.

60. False. Overvalued ideas rather than delusions are the norm.

61. True.

62. False. Delusional jealousy can present as a delusion, but also as an overvalued idea, anxious state or depressed affect.

63. True.

64. True.

Paper 2
Answers

65. False. In déjà vu, there is not an alteration of memory, but a disturbance in the feelings of familiarity associated with previously experienced situations.

66. True.

67. True.

68. False. That is the case in jamais vu.

69. True.

70. True.

71. False.

72. True.

73. True. Identifying paramnesias are déjà vu and jamais vu.

74. False. Phantom limb is a distortion of the body image (paraschemazia).

75. False. Jamais vu and déjà vu are normal phenomena, although they can be more frequent in temporal lobe epilepsy or cerebrovascular disorder.

76. True.

77. True.

78. False. This is déjà vu.

79. True.

80. False. This is one of Bleuler's primary symptoms of schizophrenia. The other three are incongruence of affect, autism (meaning preference for the inner world) and ambivalence.

81. False. Overinclusiveness is typical of schizophrenic thought disorder, and involves diffuse limits between the boundaries of concepts. It is not a first rank symptom.

Paper 2
Answers

82. False. Only those auditory hallucinations that speak out loud the patient's thoughts, or consist of running commentaries of the patient's actions, or argue amongst themselves are considered first rank symptoms.

83. True.

84. True.

85. True.

86. True.

87. False. They can be present in other processes, such as mania.

88. False. First rank symptoms are usually regarded as complementary to other signs and symptoms in establishing the diagnosis of schizophrenia.

89. False.

90. False. They also apply in other cultural settings.

91. False. The only delusions classified as first rank symptoms are delusional perceptions.

92. True.

93. True. There are, however, subtle differences; gedankenlautwerden and audible thoughts are heard at the same time they are thought, whereas écho de pensées are experienced as an echo, with a certain delay.

94. True. Thoughts that actually arise from within the self are attributed to an external agency.

95. False.

96. True.

97. False. Somatic passivity is a disturbance of thought whereas haptic hallucination is a disturbance of perception; however, a haptic or somatic hallucination may be explained in the context of somatic passivity.

98. False. It is actually a primary criterion.

99. False. Delusions and hallucinations are considered secondary criteria.

100. False.

101. False. They are first rank symptoms in Schneider's classification.

102. True.

103. False.

104. True. Bleuler's 'four As' are loosening of associations, ambivalence, autism and incongruity of affect.

105. False. Neither of the two is true.

Paper 3
Questions

Paper 3
Questions

1. Primary symptoms of schizophrenia, according to Bleuler include autism, mutism and catatonic phenomena.

2. According to Bleuler, inappropriate affect and disorganised behaviour have more importance than auditory hallucinations in establishing a diagnosis of schizophrenia.

3. The concept of overinclusive thinking was introduced by Bleuler.

4. A characteristic inability to preserve the boundaries of a concept is known as concrete thinking.

5. The term overinclusive thinking was coined by Cameron, and refers to the difficulties in respecting conceptual boundaries seen in schizophrenia.

6. Overinclusive thinking is typically seen in mania.

7. Overinclusive thinking can be classified as a form of loosening of associations.

8. Asyndesis is seen in formal thought disorder, and it involves lack of adequate connections between thoughts.

9. Overinclusive thinking is a first rank symptom of schizophrenia.

10. Overinclusive thinking can be measured using sorting tests.

11. Goldstein proposed the term concrete thinking as a difficulty in managing abstract concepts.

12. Thought blocking consists of the sudden interruption of the chain of thought, without explanation.

13. A patient who complains that an external agency is stealing his thoughts presents a classical example of thought blocking.

14. Thought blocking is, most of the time, caused by distraction.

15. Thought blocking is a first rank symptom of schizophrenia.

16. Bleuler considered thought blocking as a paramount symptom in establishing the diagnosis of schizophrenic illness.

17. It can be difficult to establish the difference between thought blocking and epileptic absences.

18. Thought block and attention deficit can be difficult to differentiate.

19. Thought blocking occurs typically in borderline states and anorexia nervosa.

20. Schizophrenic speech derives from an abnormality in language rather than from any alteration in thought.

21. Loosening of associations is only seen in schizophrenia.

22. Thought disorder can be revealed by an inappropriate use of grammar, words and concepts.

23. Tangentiality and circumstantiality are equivalent terms.

24. A patient who shows excessive difficulties with spelling of common words and delusions of reference is quite likely to be suffering from formal thought disorder.

25. Bleuler considered that the inability to form appropriate connections between thoughts was not as important as hallucinations and delusions in schizophrenia.

26. Asyndesis is the inability to preserve conceptual boundaries, and may be a feature of formal thought disorder.

27. Flight of ideas, perseveration and loosening of associations can combine in formal thought disorder.

28. A patient presenting with obsessions and paranoid ideas presents formal thought disorder.

29. Derailment, loss of goal in speech, illogicality, poor content of speech and tangentiality are features of formal thought disorder described by Andreasen.

30. In formal thought disorder, the concept of derailment involves the failure in reaching a logical conclusion following coherent associations of thoughts.

Paper 3
Questions

31. The style of speech typically seen in schizophrenic patients that contains statements that are vague, stereotyped, over-abstract or over-concrete and that convey little information is called tangential thought.

32. Vorbeireden and word salad are equivalent terms.

33. Formal thought disorder is usually seen in affective psychosis.

34. Tardive dyskinesia is a catatonic phenomenon.

35. Catatonia, by definition, is a state of increased muscular tone that is not abolished by voluntary movements.

36. Stereotypy is an abnormality of speech in which phrasal constructions become repetitive and lacking direct meaning.

37. Automatic obedience is classified under catatonic phenomena.

38. Commenting on the affect of the patient can enhance disclosure in the interview.

39. The term stupor refers to mutism and akinesia in a state of reduced level of consciousness that is quite suggestive of depression.

40. Cataplexy is a catatonic phenomenon that can be observed in schizophrenia.

41. Tardive dyskinesia only appears secondary to neuroleptic medication.

42. Echolalia consists of the inappropriate repetition of words by the patient that have been pronounced by someone else.

43. Echopraxia involves the patient committing impulsively an action when asked by someone, without considering the consequences.

44. Both waxy flexibility and psychological pillow are considered catatonic phenomena.

45. The neuroleptic malignant syndrome is one of the catatonic phenomena.

46. Magical undoing is a feature of anancastic personality disorder.

47. Stupor has been defined as the lack of relational functions.

48. "Schnauzkrampf" is a German term that refers to an alteration of volition typically seen in schizophrenia.

49. Negativism involves having negative cognitions about the future.

50. In ambitendency, negativism and automatic obedience alternate.

51. Obstruction is a technique used in cognitive psychotherapy to prevent painful thoughts from lingering in the patient's consciousness.

52. Obstruction and thought blocking can be considered analogous terms.

53. Catatonic phenomena in schizophrenia can be attributed to an underlying neurological abnormality.

54. The German term 'mitgehen' denotes excessive resistance to passive movements, and can be seen in catatonic schizophrenia.

55. The term catatonic schizophrenia was coined by Kraepeling.

56. Mannerisms are typically involuntary.

57. Stereotypy denotes the adoption of a bizarre posture for lengthy periods of time.

58. Narcolepsy is characterised by irresistible attacks of sleep that typically last for hours.

59. Catalepsy and hypnagogic hallucinations constitute the classical picture of narcolepsy.

60. Hypnagogic hallucinations occur from sleep into wakefulness.

61. Hypnopompic hallucinations usually denote functional pathology.

Paper 3
Questions

62. The onset of narcolepsy normally occurs in the fourth decade of life.

63. In narcolepsy, the association of cataplexy, sleep paralysis and hypnagogic hallucinations is seen.

64. Structural changes in certain hypothalamic regions are a common finding in subjects with narcolepsy.

65. Hypnagogic hallucinations are most frequently of a visual nature.

66. The term sleep paralysis refers to the inability to move in the transition between sleep and wakefulness.

67. Hypnagogic hallucinations are usually distressing for the subject, and almost invariably require pharmacological treatment.

68. Hypnopompic hallucinations occur in the transition from wakefulness to sleep.

69. In narcolepsy, the subject falls immediately into sleep phase three.

70. A delusion is, by definition, a false belief that is out of touch with the person's cultural, social and religious background, and is held with extraordinary tenacity and a subjective sense of certainty.

71. Although not characteristic of obsessive–compulsive disorder (OCD), delusions are commonly seen in this disorder.

72. A primary delusion arises from a hallucinatory experience.

73. The presence of primary delusions in a newly diagnosed case of schizophrenia is associated with a better prognosis.

74. A delusional perception is an abnormal idea that arises following a hallucinatory experience.

75. Persecutory delusions are less common than passivity phenomena in schizophrenia.

76. Persecutory delusions may be seen in the clinical picture of psychotic depression.

77. The presence of paranoid delusions in a patient with illusions, Lilliputian hallucinations and gross mood disturbance favours the diagnosis of schizophrenia.

78. Morbid jealousy is always associated with overvalued ideas.

79. Othello syndrome and morbid jealousy are synonymous.

80. The presence of marital infidelity rules out, by definition, a diagnosis of morbid jealousy.

81. The presence of auditory hallucinations is quite frequent in morbid jealousy.

82. Delusional jealousy responds well to a combination of cognitive therapy and typical antipsychotics.

83. Delusional jealousy is less frequent in alcohol users than in teetotallers.

84. Delusions of infidelity are more common in women than men.

85. There is a known link between chronic traumatic encephalopathy and delusional jealousy.

86. Delusional jealousy is often associated with impotence.

87. Delusional jealousy is most commonly seen in the context of paranoid schizophrenia.

88. Delusional jealousy is rarely seen in homosexual couples.

89. Delusional jealousy is seen less frequently in cohabiters than in married couples.

90. Violence is commonly seen in delusional jealousy, and is usually directed against the perceived rival.

91. Morbid jealousy is a fairly common motivation for homicide.

92. Delusional jealousy is associated with wife battering.

Paper 3
Questions

93. In most cases of morbid jealousy, a concomitant diagnosis of schizophrenia can be made.

94. In delusional jealousy, the deluded partner is usually quite emotionally independent of the other partner.

95. From a phenomenological point of view, erotomania and nymphomania are roughly equivalent terms.

96. Old maid's insanity and erotomania have been used as synonyms.

97. Persecutory delusions are often seen in the context of erotomania.

98. Erotomania is sometimes associated with bipolar affective disorder.

99. De Clérambault's syndrome is a modality of nihilistic delusion.

100. There is usually sexual intent in de Clérambault's syndrome.

101. There is an association between de Clérambault's syndrome and paranoid schizophrenia.

102. Erotomania is one of the delusional misidentification disorders.

103. De Clérambault's syndrome is a form of communicated insanity.

104. Delusional misidentification is the essential feature in de Clérambault's syndrome.

105. Erotomania is more frequent in males in the second decade of life.

Paper 3
Answers

Paper 3
Answers

1. False.

2. True.

3. False. Cameron introduced the concept of overinclusive thinking.

4. False. Concrete thinking refers to the inability to manage abstract concepts. The definition given corresponds to overinclusive thinking.

5. True.

6. False.

7. True.

8. True.

9. False.

10. True.

11. True.

12. True.

13. False. This is thought withdrawal.

14. False. On introspection, a patient cannot explain what caused this interruption in the flow of thought.

15. False.

16. False.

17. True. In both cases, the patient finds no explanation for that particular experience.

18. True.

19. False.

20. False.

21. False. It can be seen in other disorders, such as acute manic state.

22. True.

23. False.

24. False. A delusional state does not necessarily involve formal thought disorder.

25. False. He considered loosening of associations as a primary symptom, and hallucinations and delusions as secondary symptoms.

26. True. It was described by Cameron when he introduced the concept of overinclusive thinking.

27. True.

28. False.

29. True. So are neologisms and thought block, but those mentioned in the question are more frequent.

30. False. That is loss of goal rather than derailment. In derailment, the stream of thought falls onto a different line that can be of little or no relevance.

31. False. That form of thought has been termed poverty of content of speech by Andreasen. Tangentiality refers to answering questions in an irrelevant manner that denotes that the question has been understood.

32. False. "Vorbeideren" is talking past the point. In word salad, the speech is a succession of words without any structure, becoming not understandable.

33. False. Is typically seen in schizophrenia.

34. False. Tardive dyskinesia is an extrapyramidal effect.

35. False. That definition corresponds to extrapyramidal reaction. In catatonia, there is an increase in muscular tone, but this is eliminated with voluntary movements.

Paper 3
Answers

36. False. Stereotypy refers to a catatonic phenomenon in which a bizarre posture may be adopted for hours.

37. True.

38. True.

39. False. Mutism presents in a state of full consciousness.

40. False. Cataplexy refers to the sudden loss of muscle tone that occurs typically in narcolepsy, and can be provoked by strong emotion.

41. False. It has been described to be secondary to other medications (i.e., antidepressants) but can also be unrelated to any medication.

42. True.

43. False. Echopraxia refers to the repetition of an action just performed by another person.

44. True.

45. True.

46. False. It is a defence mechanism in OCD.

47. True. Relational functions refer to speech and movement.

48. False. It is equivalent to the term grimacing, which involves an abnormal facial expression in which the lips and nose are drawn together in a pout.

49. False. Negativism is a catatonic phenomenon and refers to the lack of compliance shown by the patient to execute motor commands.

50. True. A patient who begins a movement (for instance, shaking hands) and then withdraws is showing ambitendency.

51. False. It is a catatonic phenomenon in which the flow of action is suddenly interrupted.

52. True. Obstruction affects the flow of action whereas thought blocking affects the flow of thought.

Paper 3
Answers

53. True. In fact, Cutting (1985) attributed them to hemispheric imbalance.

54. False. Actually 'mitgehen' denotes excessive compliance (going with).

55. False. Kahlbaum described it in 1873.

56. False. They are also called idiosyncratic voluntary movements and are odd voluntary movements or patterns of behaviour.

57. True. Stereotypy is a catatonic feature.

58. False. The duration of the attacks is typically 10–15 minutes.

59. False. Catalepsy is one of the catatonic phenomena in which the body maintains a given posture for a certain period of time. Cataplexy is seen in narcolepsy and involves a sudden loss of muscle tone, and can be triggered by strong emotion.

60. False. Hypnagogic hallucinations occur in the transition from wakefulness into sleep.

61. False. Hypnopompic and hypnagogic hallucinations occur with relative frequency in normality.

62. False. It normally begins in adolescence and persists throughout adult life.

63. True.

64. False. There are usually no structural changes.

65. False. They are typically auditory.

66. True.

67. False. They are normal phenomena.

68. False.

69. False. It is REM sleep or phase five.

Paper 3
Answers

70. True.

71. False.

72. False. By definition, a primary delusion arises *de novo* and, hence, is not connected to any psychopathological abnormality.

73. False. Neither primary delusions nor first rank symptoms have prognostic value.

74. False. A delusional perception is formed after a normal perception that is given a delusional explanation.

75. False. Delusions of persecution are the most common delusions.

76. True. Persecutory delusions are commonly seen in schizophrenia and other psychotic states, as well as affective and organic disorders.

77. False. The clinical picture described corresponds to delirium tremens.

78. False. Actually morbid jealousy can present in the form of delusions, overvalued ideas or anxiety.

79. True.

80. False. The important factor is the presence of abnormal ideas that do not correspond with the evidence available to the subject.

81. False. Morbid jealousy typically presents as a false, isolated belief in the absence of other psychopathology.

82. False. The abnormal ideas in delusional jealousy tend to be very resistant to treatment, and usually run a chronic course.

83. False. There is a link between delusional jealousy and alcohol abuse (Shresta et al., 1985)

84. False. It is more common in men.

85. True. Lishman (1997) describes a connection between the punch-drunk syndrome seen in boxers and delusional jealousy.

Paper 3
Answers

86. True.

87. False.

88. False. It is more frequent amongst the homosexual population.

89. False. Delusions of infidelity are more frequent in couples who lack a legal sanction.

90. False. Although there is a strong association of violence in delusional jealousy, this is typically directed towards the partner instead of the suspected lover.

91. True.

92. True.

93. False.

94. False. The deluded person is usually very emotionally attached and sometimes dependant upon the victim.

95. False. Nymphomania is a behavioural and emotional abnormality regarding sexual conduct, whereas erotomania is a delusional state.

96. True. The former term was introduced by Hart (1921).

97. True.

98. True.

99. False. De Clérambault's syndrome is a type of erotomania in which the sufferer (typically female) believes that a person, who is usually older and of higher social status, is in love with her and she loves him in return.

100. False. Sexual intention is typically absent in erotomania.

101. True. Also associated with bipolar affective disorder.

102. False. Only Capgras, Frégoli, intermetamorphosis and subjective doubles are delusional misidentifications.

Paper 3
Answers

103. False. The term communicated insanity refers to folie á deux and related phenomena.

104. False.

105. False. It is commoner in females. (Old maid's insanity).

Paper 4
Questions

Paper 4
Questions

1. In the forensic setting, the male patients suffering from de Clérambault's syndrome outnumber female patients.

2. Delusional misidentification is a disorder of face processing.

3. Prosopagnosia is a delusional misidentification.

4. In Capgras' syndrome, the patient believes that some close relative or friend has been replaced by an impostor.

5. Capgras' syndrome is a hallucinatory phenomenon.

6. The name of Reboul-Lachaux is related to the syndrome of Frégoli.

7. In Frégoli syndrome, the person recognises familiar people in strangers.

8. Frégoli syndrome is a hallucinatory state.

9. In Capgras' syndrome, the patient has nihilistic delusions associated with elated mood.

10. Capgras' syndrome and Frégoli syndrome are not very different.

11. In Frégoli syndrome, the patient believes that another person has been transformed into his own self.

12. The syndrome of intermetamorphosis is an identifying paramnesia.

13. In the syndrome of intermetamorphosis, the subject believes that a familiar person has been transformed into another person.

14. There is a link between Capgras' syndrome and schizophrenia.

15. Capgras' syndrome arises from a delusional percept.

16. Capgras' syndrome involves the illusion that a person has been replaced by a double.

17. Frégoli syndrome is a delusional disorder that involves the belief that a familiar person who persecutes the patient has taken a different appearance.

18. The primary cause of delusional misidentification is organic process.

19. In the initial phases of chronic alcoholic hallucinosis, auditory hallucinations are characteristically fragmented.

20. Ambivalence is a classical symptom of normal grief.

21. Cotard's syndrome and 'illusion des sosies' are synonymous.

22. Cotard's syndrome is a nihilistic delusional disorder.

23. The presence of Cotard's syndrome favours a diagnosis of functional disorder against an organic process.

24. Nihilistic delusions are delusions of unworthiness.

25. The prevalent psychopathological feature of Cotard's syndrome is hypochondriacal delusions.

26. Ekbom syndrome is a delusion of infestation.

27. Repetitive acts precede intrusive thoughts in OCD.

28. Prader–Willy syndrome and Klein–Levin syndrome are associated with hyperphagia.

29. In hebephrenic schizophrenia, hallucinations and delusions are not prominent.

30. Cotard's syndrome is seen in OCD.

31. Symptoms in Ganser syndrome include the presence of the grasp reflex.

32. Night terror is a dissociative phenomenon.

33. Bouffe delirante is a culture-bound syndrome involving violent outbursts.

Paper 4
Questions

34. In Ekbom syndrome, the patient thinks he is contaminated with microscopic organisms.

35. Ekbom syndrome can involve overvalued ideas.

36. Ekbom syndrome has not been described in combination with schizophrenia.

37. Couvade's syndrome is a delusional state.

38. In Couvade's syndrome, the husband of a pregnant woman presents symptoms related to his wife's pregnancy.

39. The most important factor in establishing a diagnosis of Couvade's syndrome is the presence of pseudo-obstetric symptoms in the husband.

40. The symptoms in Couvade's syndrome are quite specific of that disorder.

41. In Couvade's syndrome, the husband of a pregnant lady holds the erroneous belief that he is also pregnant.

42. Briquet's syndrome is a delusional state.

43. Conversion disorder and Briquet's syndrome have been used as synonymous.

44. Briquet's disorder involves the presence of obstetrics symptoms in the partner of a pregnant woman.

45. Somatisation disorder and Briquet's syndrome are equivalent terms.

46. Autoscopy involves seeing oneself in the external space, viewed from within one's own body.

47. Autoscopy is frequently seen in schizophrenia.

48. There is a link between narcissism and autoscopy.

49. Visual imagery is associated to autoscopy.

Paper 4
Questions

50. Autoscopy is characteristically a hallucinatory phenomenon.

51. The phenomenon described as 'phantom mirror image' and autoscopy differ in the lack of insight in the subject.

52. In depression, there is reduced REM latency.

53. Dichotomous thinking is a cognitive distortion in depression.

54. Erotomania is a misidentification syndrome.

55. An overinclusion mechanism is involved in flight of ideas.

56. Cataplexy is a catatonic symptom.

57. Autoscopy is usually seen in Capgras' syndrome.

58. Autoscopy is a form of extracampine hallucination.

59. In functional hallucinations, an external stimulus is necessary to provoke a hallucination in the same sensory modality.

60. In schizophrenia, a visual stimulus can produce a functional auditory hallucination.

61. The presence of functional hallucinations helps to differentiate schizophrenia from organic psychosis.

62. Pseudohallucinations occur in the external subjective space.

63. Pseudohallucinations can be evoked in delirium tremens.

64. Pseudohallucinations are not subjectively different from normal perceptions.

65. Pseudohallucinations occur in normal people.

66. Pseudohallucinations are commonly described in schizophrenia.

67. In normal bereavement, the occurrence of pseudohallucinations is rare.

Paper 4
Questions

68. A person suffering from pseudohallucinations regards these phenomena as abnormal.

69. Illusions, hallucinations and pseudohallucinations have in common the perception of unreal objects.

70. An illusion involves the perception of an object that is not there.

71. Completion illusions become clearer when attention is focused upon them.

72. Affect illusions are independent of the prevailing mood state.

73. Affect illusions become clearer when the subject directs attention to them.

74. Pareidolia is induced by psychomimetic drugs.

75. Direct entry into REM sleep is characteristic of narcolepsy.

76. Bleuler's fundamental symptoms of schizophrenia include incongruity of affect.

77. Koro is a psychotic disorder.

78. Primary delusions are more common in acute schizophrenia than in chronic schizophrenia.

79. In chronic alcoholic hallucinosis, auditory hallucinations are characteristically fragmented to start with.

80. Munchausen's patients confabulate.

81. OCD is associated to de Clérambault's syndrome.

82. Pareidolic illusions are banished under close attention.

83. Pareidolic illusions are independent of imagination.

84. Pareidolic illusions are functional hallucinations.

85. Day dreaming and pareidolia are equivalent terms.

86. Panoramic memory is involved in temporal lobe epilepsy.

87. Confabulation is fluent lying.

88. Catatonic symptoms are found in 20% of hebephrenics.

89. In depression, there is abnormality in time perception.

90. Confabulation is associated with organic states.

91. Night terrors are associated with dissociative disorders.

92. Patients with mania often have some sadness.

93. Olfactory hallucinations are characteristically experienced in cocaine withdrawal.

94. In confabulation, there is usually a decreased level of consciousness.

95. In confabulation of embarrassment, the subject tries to cover up an embarrassing event with a falsified memory.

96. In Korsakov's syndrome, confabulation is typical of the later stages of the process.

97. Suggestibility is associated with confabulation.

98. Confabulation occurs in dementia.

99. Tangentiality is a good indicator of imminent schizophrenia relapse.

100. Confabulation occurs in schizophrenia.

101. Sensory distortions occur exclusively in organic states.

102. Hyperacusis and visual hyperaesthesia are examples of pseudohallucinations.

103. Forced thinking before a convulsion is characteristic of temporal lobe epilepsy.

Paper 4
Questions

104. Dysmegalopsia is best described as a hallucinatory phenomenon.

105. Sensory distortions are abnormal perceptions.

Paper 4
Answers

Paper 4
Answers

1. True. Although this disorder is more common in females.

2. True.

3. False. It is the inability to recognise faces.

4. True.

5. False. The underlying psychopathological alteration is a delusion.

6. False. Reboul-Lachaux and Capgras described the syndrome with the former name.

7. True.

8. False. Is a delusional state.

9. False. Capgras' syndrome is a delusional misidentification that involves a double substituting a familiar person.

10. True. Both are delusional misidentifications.

11. False. That description corresponds to the syndrome of subjective doubles.

12. False. Identifying paramnesias are déjà vu and related experiences.

13. True.

14. True. It is also associated to organic psychosis and bipolar disorder.

15. True. A normal perception is given a delusional meaning.

16. False. It is not an illusion but a delusion.

17. True.

18. False. It is usually schizophrenia; it is also linked to affective psychosis.

19. True. Auditory hallucinations are usually simple words or small sentences in organic states, although they can become very elaborate in alcoholic hallucinosis.

20. False.

21. False. The term 'illusion des sosies' (illusion of doubles) refers to Capgras' syndrome. The French term for Cotard's syndrome is 'délire de negation'.

22. True.

23. False. Cotard's syndrome can be also seen in organic processes.

24. False. Nihilistic delusions involve negation.

25. True. The association of hypochondriacal and nihilistic delusions in psychotic depression consitiutes Cotard's syndrome.

26. True.

27. False.

28. True.

29. True.

30. False.

31. False. The four features of Ganser syndrome are: 1) approximate answers; 2) psychogenic physical symptoms; 3) hallucinations; and 4) apparent clouding of consciousness. It is classified as a dissociative disorder.

32. False.

33. False. Bouffe delirante is a French term more or less equivalent to acute delusional state.

34. False. The belief typically involves macroscopic organisms.

35. True. The syndrome may present as a delusion, overvalued idea or hallucinatory state (usually tactile).

Paper 4
Answers

36. False. It is typically seen in psychotic depression.

37. False. It is a conversion syndrome.

38. True.

39. False. It is the chronological relationship of symptoms with the wife's pregnancy.

40. False. Symptoms are rather unspecific, such as anxiety, tension, insomnia, nausea and vomiting, toothache.

41. False. It is not a delusional state, but a conversion syndrome of the husband's anxiety into somatic symptoms.

42. False. It is a term used to define somatisation disorder, which is characterised by multiple and frequently changing somatic complaints that do not appear to be due to physical disorder.

43. False. Briquet's syndrome is synonymous of somatisation disorder. A conversion disorder involves the presence of psychogenic symptoms (usually pseudoneurological)

44. False. That is Couvade's syndrome.

45. True.

46. True.

47. False. It is rare, and is most commonly seen in depression.

48. True.

49. True.

50. False. It is an alteration of self-perception and can present as a pseudohallucination.

51. False. Both terms are synonymous.

52. True.

53. True.

Paper 4
Answers

54. False.

55. True. Overinclusion was described by Cameron as the inability to preserve the boundaries of a concept.

56. False.

57. False. Autoscopy is an alteration of unity of the self and Capgras' syndrome is a delusional misidentification.

58. False. Extracampine hallucinations are experienced outside the limits of the sensory field.

59. True.

60. False. The event described is a reflex hallucination; functional hallucinations are in the same modality as the provoking normal percept.

61. False. Neither functional nor reflex hallucinations have greater diagnostic significance.

62. False. Pseudohallucinations occur in the internal subjective space.

63. False. Pseudohallucinations cannot be evoked.

64. False.

65. True.

66. True.

67. False.

68. True.

69. True.

70. True.

71. False. Completion illusions depend on inattention; this is what happens when we miss the misprints in the newspapers. As soon as attention is focused on them, the error becomes clear.

Paper 4
Answers

72. False.

73. False.

74. True.

75. True.

76. True.

77. False. It is classified as an anxiety disorder; it is accompanied by the belief that the penis will sink into the abdomen and result in death. More frequently seen in South East Asia.

78. True.

79. True. Auditory hallucinations are usually simple words or small sentences in organic states, although they can become very elaborate in alcoholic hallucinosis.

80. False. Confabulation involves the replacement of a memory by fantasy. In Munchausen's, there is a tendency to exaggerate or lie about medical symptoms, and is associated with the term pseudologia fantastica.

81. False.

82. False.

83. False. They involve a mixture of perception and imagination.

84. False.

85. False.

86. True. Panoramic recall is a rapid re-enactment of long periods in the patient's life.

87. False.

88. True.

89. True.

Paper 4
Answers

90. True.

91. False.

92. True.

93. False. Formication is the most characteristic hallucination related to cocaine, and is a tactile hallucination.

94. False. Confabulations are falsifications of memory that are associated with organic states and occur in clear consciousness.

95. False.

96. False. Confabulation most commonly appears in the early stages of Korsakov's syndrome and gradually disappears with the deterioration of the intellectual function.

97. True.

98. True.

99. False.

100. True.

101. False.

102. False. They are sensory distortions in which the intensity of a perception is heightened.

103. False. Forced thinking occurs in frontopolar seizures.

104. False. It is a sensory distortion.

105. True. In sensory distortions, the intensity or quality of a perception is altered.

Paper 5
Questions

Paper 5
Questions

1. Sensory distortions are perceptions without an object.

2. In derealisation, there is a sensory distortion.

3. Micropsia involves seeing objects smaller on one side than the other.

4. In splitting of perception, the subject fails to form the normal connections between two or more perceptions.

5. Stupor is defined by the absence of action and speech in clear consciousness.

6. Akinesis and mutism occur in stupor.

7. In a mute and akinetic patient with a severely reduced level of consciousness, the most likely diagnosis is stupor.

8. An autochthonous delusion is egosyntonic.

9. Stupor is almost exclusively seen in schizophrenia.

10. Total absence of voluntary movements is seen in stupor.

11. Stupor can be seen in neuroleptic malignant syndrome.

12. In delirium tremens, the level of consciousness is preserved.

13. A high level of arousal can be seen in delirium tremens.

14. The onset of delirium tremens usually occurs in the first 24 hours after the last drink.

15. Lilliputian hallucinations are typical of delirium tremens.

16. In delirium tremens, there are changes in the affective state.

17. Illusions can occur in delirium tremens.

18. Suggestibility is present in delirium tremens.

19. Delusions can be a prominent feature in delirium tremens.

20. Visual hallucinations are a prominent feature of delirium tremens.

21. The terms haptic and hygric hallucinations are synonymous.

22. Hallucinations of bodily sensations are common in schizophrenia.

23. Hallucinations of bodily sensations are associated with delusions.

24. Ekbom's syndrome and formication are synonymous terms.

25. Formication is seen in alcohol withdrawal.

26. Formication is characteristically associated with cocaine addiction.

27. Ekbom's syndrome is a hallucinatory state.

28. Latah is a delusional disorder.

29. In koro, a disorder of body image exists.

30. An overinclusion mechanism is involved in flight of ideas.

31. Amok is typically found in Malaysia.

32. The belief that the penis will shrink into the abdomen is the cardinal feature of windigo.

33. Tangentiality is pathognomonic of schizophrenia.

34. Pareidolic illusions disappear on concentrating.

35. Erotomania is seen in Cotard's syndrome.

36. Evil eye is characteristically seen in Haiti.

37. In windigo, a phobic state is seen.

38. Amok is a phobic state seen in Malaysia.

39. Alcoholic hallucinosis and delirium tremens are synonymous terms.

Paper 5
Questions

40. In alcoholic hallucinosis, there is decreased level of consciousness.

41. Loosening of associations and derailment are very different terms.

42. In depersonalisation, people around you feel 'unreal'.

43. Alcoholic hallucinosis occurs typically in individuals who have been drinking excessively over several years.

44. Silence can enhance disclosure in the interview.

45. Alcoholic hallucinosis is currently classified as a schizophrenic illness released by alcohol consumption.

46. In alcoholic hallucinosis, the auditory hallucinations are initially elementary.

47. Third-person auditory hallucinations are seen in alcoholic hallucinosis.

48. In alcoholic hallucinosis, the patient may respond to hallucinatory commands.

49. In auditory hallucinosis, primary delusions occur.

50. Alcoholic hallucinations typically occur in the withdrawal phase of alcohol dependence.

51. In stereotypy, the movement is meaningless and not repetitive.

52. Rotational vertigo is an anxiety symptom.

53. Lack of empathy is a feature of alexithymia.

54. Auditory hallucinations in alcoholic hallucinosis can lead to persecutory delusions.

55. In acute schizophrenia, the patient usually retains insight.

56. Mannerisms are non-purposeful repetitive movements.

57. There are changes in tactile sensation in depersonalisation.

58. The auditory hallucinations seen in alcoholic hallucinosis are structured and persistent.

59. An alcoholic hallucinosis, primary delusions occur.

60. Alexithymia is the inability to write.

61. Alcoholic hallucinosis usually has a bad prognosis despite alcohol abstinence.

62. Tics are rapid voluntary and stereotyped movements that cannot be voluntarily repeated by the individual.

63. Gilles de la Tourette usually commences with complex tics before the age of 16 years.

64. Vocalizations are common in Tourette's syndrome.

65. Coprolalia is rarely seen in Gilles de la Tourette.

66. Coprophagia is a feature of Gilles de la Tourette.

67. Tics are more likely to occur under stress.

68. Adult sufferers of Gilles de la Tourette present greater OCD features than controls.

69. Adult sufferers of Tourette's syndrome present greater incidence of depression than controls.

70. Gilles de la Tourette is more frequent in females.

71. Tics and forced vocalizations are central features in Gilles de la Tourette.

72. Visual hallucinations tend to occur in functional states.

73. Elementary thoughts can be audible thoughts.

74. Obsessional thoughts can be pleasurable.

75. Visual hallucinations occur in epilepsy.

Paper 5
Questions

76. Homonymous hemianopia can be accompanied by visual hallucinations.

77. Visual hallucinations occur in Alzheimer's disease.

78. Visual perceptual disturbances occur in up to 30% of psychogeriatric patients.

79. Ocular pathology in elderly patients is strongly associated with visual hallucinations.

80. Visual hallucinations are less frequent in glue sniffing.

81. Visual hallucinations are uncommon in schizophrenia.

82. In schizophrenia, visual hallucinations are commonly associated with visual pseudohallucinations.

83. Visual hallucinations occur in uncomplicated affective states.

84. In the Charles Bonnet syndrome, visual hallucinations occur in the context of delirium.

85. Lilliputian hallucinations are a characteristic feature of delirium tremens.

86. Visual illusions occur in delirium tremens.

87. Autoscopy is an abnormality of visual perception.

88. The presence of visual hallucinations strongly suggests organic pathology.

89. Shock and denial are characteristic of the immediate experience of loss.

90. The presentation of symptoms of the last illness of the deceased in a bereaved person is consistent with normal grief reaction.

91. Agitated depression is seen in normal grief.

92. Marked psychomotor retardation is seen in abnormal grief reaction.

93. Delay in the presentation of a grief reaction is seen in abnormal grief.

94. Illusions or hallucinations of the deceased person are indicative of abnormal grief reaction.

95. Grief reactions can be seen in babies who lose a parent even before the development of attachment behaviour.

96. Autonomic symptoms are seen in the mourning phase of normal grief.

97. The stunned phase of normal grief lasts up to 2 months.

98. Normal grief reaction has a typical duration of 6 months.

99. Elementary hallucinations can occur in the form of thought echo.

100. Phobic avoidance of things related to the deceased is seen in normal grief.

101. One of the dimensions of insight involves the ability to re-label unusual mental events as pathological.

102. In schizophrenia, insight is usually preserved.

103. In acutely manic patients, improvement in insight does correlate with improvement in other symptoms.

104. Insight is a multifaceted phenomenon.

105. From a practical point of view, the most important aspect of insight is the ability to classify abnormal experiences as pathological.

Paper 5
Answers

Paper 5
Answers

1. False. Hallucinations are perceptions without an object.

2. True. There is a change in the feeling of reality of the perceptual field.

3. False. That is dysmegalopsia; micropsia is seeing objects smaller than their actual size.

4. True. This is a rare phenomenon occasionally seen in schizophrenia; usually perceptions in different modalities that are normally integrated are perceived as separate and even conflicting events. Splitting of perception is a sensory distortion.

5. True.

6. True.

7. False. Stupor occurs in clear consciousness.

8. True. The individual fails to see them as a problem and integrates them into his identity.

9. False. It also occurs in depression, mania and dissociative states.

10. True.

11. True.

12. False. The cardinal features of delirium tremens are decreased level of consciousness, perceptual abnormalities and disturbances in mood.

13. True. Despite this, the level of consciousness is decreased and the subject only has fluctuating awareness of his surroundings.

14. False. It normally occurs from the second to the seventh day after ceasing to drink.

15. True.

16. True. The mood in delirium tremens is typically described as being of terror with an admixture of jocularity.

Paper 5
Answers

17. True. These are typically prodromal to hallucinations.

18. True. Visual illusions and hallucinations can be induced by suggestion.

19. True.

20. True.

21. False. Both are hallucinations of bodily sensation, but haptic refers to a hallucination of touch whereas hygric refers to a hallucination of perception of fluid.

22. True.

23. True. They are often associated with delusions of control.

24. False. Formication refers to a bodily hallucination of little insects crawling over or under one's skin, whereas Ekbom's syndrome refers to a delusion of infestation. Although frequently seen together, they are not synonymous terms.

25. True.

26. True.

27. False. It is a delusion of infestation.

28. False. It is best described as a conversion disorder.

29. True.

30. True. Overinclusion was described by Cameron as the inability to preserve the boundaries of a concept.

31. True.

32. False. It is characteristic of koro.

33. False.

34. False.

35. False.

36. False. North Africa and Mexico.

37. False. It is a depressive state following fears of engaging in cannibalism seen in Native Canadians.

38. False. It is a dissociative state.

39. False. Cardinal features of alcoholic hallucinosis include auditory hallucinations in clear consciousness without autonomic hyperactivity.

40. False.

41. False. In derailment there is a breakdown in associations.

42. False.

43. True.

44. True.

45. False. It is classified in ICD-10 as a psychotic state induced by alcohol.

46. True.

47. True.

48. True.

49. False. Although delusions can be present in alcoholic hallucinosis, these are typically secondary to auditory hallucinations.

50. False. Delirium tremens is more typical of alcohol withdrawal.

51. False. Stereotypy involves adopting an uncomfortable posture for long periods of time. It should not be confused with stereotyped movements, that are repeated movements without significance. The difference with mannerisms is that the latter are usually meaningful.

Paper 5
Answers

52. False. However, dizziness may be provoked by hyperventilation in an anxious state.

53. True. Alexithymia is the inability to identify, define and discriminate between emotions. Empathy is the sensitivity to the feelings of others.

54. True.

55. False.

56. False. Mannerisms appear to have functional significance.

57. True. There can be changes in all perceptual modalities.

58. True.

59. False.

60. False. Alexithymia refers to difficulty in expressing affect and emotions. There is diminished fantasy and abstract thinking. It is seen in psychosomatic disorders, somatoform disorders, psychogenic pain disorders, substance misuse, PTSD, masked depression, neurosis and disorders of sexual conduct.

61. False.

62. False. Tics are involuntary, but they can usually be faithfully reproduced by the subject.

63. False. Although the onset of Gilles de la Tourette is usually between the ages of 5 and 8 years, it typically commences with simple tics that become more complex as the process progresses.

64. True.

65. False.

66. False.

67. True.

68. True.

69. True.

70. False.

71. True.

72. False.

73. False.

74. False. Obsessional thoughts are egodystonic, and hence found repulsive and resisted by the subject.

75. True.

76. True. Hemianopia is the loss of the same half of the visual field in both eyes.

77. True. Although more characteristic of Lewy body dementia, visual hallucinations have also been described in multi-infarct dementia, and Huntington's chorea.

78. True.

79. True.

80. False.

81. True.

82. True.

83. False.

84. False. Charles Bonnet syndrome is characterised by complex visual hallucinations associated with impaired vision in the absence of other psychopathology.

85. True.

86. True.

87. True. It involves seeing oneself in the external space.

Paper 5
Answers

88. True.

89. True.

90. False.

91. False.

92. True.

93. True.

94. False. These can be seen in normal bereavement.

95. False.

96. True.

97. False. This initial phase lasts from a few hours to 2 weeks.

98. True.

99. False. Elementary hallucinations are unstructured sounds in the auditory modality, flashes of light or colour in the visual modality.

100. False.

101. True. The other two are the recognition that one has a mental illness and the compliance with treatment.

102. False.

103. False.

104. True.

105. False. One could argue that the single most important aspect of insight is adherence to treatment.